A Practical Book

# Pharmacognosy and Phytochemistry

## CONTENTS

## Preface

Pharmaceutical sciences, especially when it comes to natural products, need a strict and organized way of doing things in the lab. Standardized methods are very important for making sure that herbal drugs and other natural product-derived pharmaceuticals are safe, effective, pure, and of good quality. Without these kinds of established protocols, it can be hard for doctors to use and accept manufactured medications in their practice. This experiment delineates a comprehensive range of practical methodologies, including microscopic and morphological characterization, the isolation and analysis of bioactive phytoconstituents, various extraction techniques, advanced chromatographic and spectrophotometric analyses, quantitative estimations, bioactivity screenings, fundamental molecular biology protocols, and assessments of pharmaceutical formulation and quality control. Each section combines theoretical foundations with step-by-step instructions, emphasizing important factors, required tools, chemical reagents, and safety precautions. This detailed guide is meant to give you a solid framework for hands-on lab work so you can learn more about natural product research and drug development.

**Authors**

# EXPERIMENT No: 01

**Object:** Microscopic and Morphological Characterization of Plant Materials by determination of Leaf Constants.

**Requirements:**

**Reagents:** Chloral hydrate solution, Glycerol ethanol solution

**Equipment:**

- Test tubes
- Boiling water bath
- Microscopic slides
- Cover slips
- Microscope (equipped with 40x objective and 6x eyepiece)
- Camera lucida
- Drawing board
- Stage micrometer

**Theory:**

Finding out the leaf constants, such as the number of stomata, the stomatal index, the number of vein islets, and the number of vein terminations, is an important pharmacognostic step. The stomatal index is a more useful diagnostic tool than the stomatal number because it stays pretty stable and isn't as affected by changes in the environment, the age of the plant, or the size of the leaf.

**Procedure:**

1. **Surface Preparation of Leaf:** A piece of a leaf that is about 5x5 mm is put into a test tube with about 5 mL of chloral hydrate solution. Then, the test tube is put in a boiling water bath for about 15 minutes, or until the leaf pieces become see-through. This chemical clearing process makes the epidermal cells and stomata easy to see under a microscope.
2. **Mounting:** A transparent leaf fragment is carefully transferred to a microscopic slide. The lower epidermis is mounted uppermost in chloral hydrate solution. To prevent the preparation from drying during observation, a small drop of glycerol ethanol solution is added to one side of the cover glass.
3. **Microscopic Examination and Drawing:** The prepared slide is examined under a

microscope utilizing a 40x objective and a 6x eyepiece, which is equipped with a microscopical drawing apparatus. A camera lucida and drawing board are arranged to facilitate drawing to scale. A square of 1 mm is delineated on the drawing board by means of a stage micrometer, providing a precise area for counting.

4. **Counting Stomata and Epidermal Cells (for Stomatal Number and Index):**

The epidermal cells and stomata are marked out in the 1 square millimeter area. We count the number of stomata in this area, making sure to include any cell that has at least half of its area inside the square. This process is done ten times for different fields of view, and the average number of stomata per square millimeter is found. To find the stomatal index, you count both the number of stomata (S) and the number of epidermal cells (E) in the same area.

5. **Counting Vein Islet Number and Vein Termination Number:**

These constants are determined by enumerating the average number of vein islets and veinlet terminations per square millimeter of the leaf surface.

**Observation Table:** Typical Leaf Constants for Identification

| **Parameter** | | | |
|---|---|---|---|
| Stomatal Index | | | |
| Vein-Islet Number (per sq. mm) | | | |
| Vein Termination Number (per sq. mm) | | | |
| Palisade Ratio | | | |

**Calculations:**

**Stomatal Index (SI):** The stomatal index is calculated as the percentage ratio of the number of stomata to the total number of epidermal cells (including stomata) in a given area.

The formula is:

$$SI = \frac{S}{S + E} X\, 100$$

Where,

S= number of stomata

E= number of epidermal cells.

**Precautions:**

1. Careful handle the glass wares.
2. Use appropriate personal protective equipment (PPE) such as lab coats and gloves.
3. Chloral hydrate, being a chemical reagent, should be handled with due care and in a well-ventilated area.

**Result:** The morphological and microscopic examination of the given plant material was observed and calculated.

# EXPERIMENT No: 02

**Object**: Determination of particle size, plant fibers, trichomes, and starch grains.

**Requirements:**

**Reagents (Lycopodium Method):** Lycopodium spores (*Lycopodium clavatum* Linn.) Suspending agent (fixed oil or glycerine: tragacanth mucilage: water 2:1:2)

**Equipment (Camera Lucida):**

- Microscope
- Stage micrometer
- Ocular micrometer
- Camera lucida (with mirror and reflecting prism)

**Equipment (Lycopodium Method):**

- Balance
- Small watch glass
- Small flexible spatula
- Microscope (with mechanical stage or counting square)

**Theory:**

The science of measuring very small sizes is important for finding microorganisms and describing crude drugs at the cellular level. This method is very helpful for finding small pieces and finding adulterants in herbal materials. The Lycopodium spore method adds to this by giving a quantitative way to analyze powdered herbal drugs. This is especially helpful when other methods of evaluation don't work as well. It makes it possible to compare a known standard to find out how many characteristic particles there are per unit weight.

**Procedure (Camera Lucida for Particle Size/Drawing):**

1. **Microscope Setup:** A camera lucida is securely attached to the microscope.
2. **Calibration:** At the desired magnification, the ocular micrometer is set up to work with a stage micrometer. This important step is figuring out the exact size of each division on the ocular micrometer scale. For example, if 10 ocular micrometer

(OM) divisions perfectly line up with 7 stage micrometer (SM) divisions at 40x magnification and each SM division is known to be 0.01 mm, then 1 OM division is equal to (7 * 0.01 mm) / 10 = 0.007 mm.

3. **Object Measurement:** After the ocular micrometer is set up, the stage micrometer is taken out and replaced with the slide that has the object you want to look at (like a plant fiber, trichome, or starch grain). After that, the object's size is measured by counting how many divisions it covers on the calibrated ocular scale.

4. **Finding the Actual Size:** To find the object's actual size, you multiply the number of ocular divisions it covers by the calibrated value of one ocular division.

5. **Drawing (Camera Lucida):** The camera lucida projects a microscopic image onto a drawing surface, which makes it possible to make accurate outline drawings that keep the object's scale and proportions correct. This ability is very useful for making detailed visual records and studying morphology.

**3. Procedure (Lycopodium Spore Method for Starch Grains/Particle Counting):**

1. **Sample Preparation**: First, the loss on drying for the powdered drug is found at 105°C. In a small watch glass, a carefully measured amount of air-dry powdered drug (e.g., 100 mg) is mixed with a carefully measured amount of Lycopodium spores (e.g., 50mg).
2. **Suspension preparation:** Use a small, flexible spatula to mix the parts together well. Add a suspending agent, like fixed oil or a 2:1:2 mixture of glycerine, tragacanth mucilage, and water. Stir the mixture for 10 minutes until it becomes a smooth paste.
3. **Dilution:** The suspension is diluted until there are about 10 to 20 Lycopodium spores in each field of view under the microscope.
4. **Microscopic Counting:** You look at the mixture under a microscope. In several fields of view (e.g., 25 different fields), the number of starch grains (or other characteristic particles) and Lycopodium spores are counted.
5. **Calculation:** To find out how many starch grains (or other particles) there are, you compare their count to the known number of visible Lycopodium spores. It is known that one milligram of Lycopodium spores has about 94,000 spores. This

method gives a numerical ratio of the different ingredients in the powdered drug, which is very useful for finding out if it has been tampered with.

**Observation**

**Table 1:** Comparison of Particle Size Determination Methods.

| Method | Principle | Primary Application | Advantages | Limitations |
|---|---|---|---|---|
| **Camera Lucida** | | | | |

**Table 2:**

| **Method** | **Principle** | **Primary Application** | **Advantages** | **Limitations** |
|---|---|---|---|---|
| | image onto a drawing surface for accurate scaling. | measurement of individual particles (length, breadth). | documentation and precise dimensional analysis of individual features. | for bulk samples, requires calibration. |
| **Lycopodium Spore Method** | Comparison of characteristic particle count in a sample to a known standard (Lycopodium spores). | Quantitative estimation of specific particles (e.g., starch grains, fibres, trichomes) per unit weight of powdered drug. | Useful for assessing quality and quantity of ingredients in powdered drugs, detecting adulteration. | Requires uniform size and distribution of reference spores; primarily for quantitative counting, not detailed morphology. |

**Precautions:**

Careful handling of chemical reagents and equipment.

**Result:** Particle size, plant fibres, trichomes, and starch grains of given sample was determined.

# EXPERIMENT No: 03

**Object:** Isolation of Curcumin from *Curcuma longa* Rhizomes.

**Requirements:**

**Reagents:**

- Ground turmeric
- Ethanol
- TLC eluent (e.g., 70:30 cyclohexane:isopropanol)
- Optional: 0.5% w/v boric acid in 1:1 ethanol:water

**Equipments:**

- Test tube and rack
- Spatula
- Glass rod
- Measuring cylinder
- Funnel
- Filter paper
- Boiling tube and rack
- Silica TLC plate
- TLC spotters/capillary tubes
- 250 mL beaker (as TLC chamber)
- Watch glass
- Tweezers

**Theory:**

- Curcumin, a significant bioactive compound in the rhizomes of Curcuma longa L. (turmeric), is esteemed for its robust antimicrobial and immunomodulatory attributes. Its isolation signifies a pivotal preliminary phase for ensuing research, purification, and the formulation of pharmaceutical products.

**Procedure (Solvent Extraction & TLC Separation):**

1. **Sample Preparation:** A quantity of 0.5 g of ground turmeric is accurately weighed and placed into a test tube.
2. **Extraction:** To the test tube, 5 mL of ethanol is added, and the mixture is gently stirred for 2-3 minutes. The mixture is then allowed to soak for a period. The selection of ethanol, or isopropanol as an alternative, represents a deliberate choice towards "greener" chemistry, prioritizing environmental and health considerations over the

potentially higher, but more hazardous, efficiency of solvents like dichloromethane and methanol. This approach reflects a growing emphasis on sustainable practices in natural product isolation.

3. **Filtration:** Following the soaking period, the mixture is stirred for a final minute. It is then filtered using a funnel equipped with fluted filter paper, collecting the filtrate in a boiling tube. Only a small volume of this filtrate is required for subsequent TLC analysis.
4. **TLC Plate Preparation:** A horizontal pencil line is lightly drawn approximately 1 cm from the bottom of a silica TLC plate, with an 'X' marked at the center of this line to designate the sample spotting location.
5. **TLC Mobile Phase Preparation:** Measure out 10 mL of the chosen TLC eluent (like a 70:30 mixture of cyclohexane and isopropanol) and pour it into a 250 mL glass beaker. It is very important to keep the solvent level below the line that marks where to spot the sample. A folded piece of filter paper that has been soaked in the eluent is put inside the TLC chamber (beaker) to act as a wick. This keeps the chamber full of solvent vapors and stops evaporation. The watch glass is then put over the beaker.
6. **Sample Spotting:** A capillary tube is used to put a small amount of the filtered turmeric extract on the "X" mark on the TLC plate. Let the spot dry completely before Moving on.
7. **TLC Development:** Using tweezers, the TLC plate is carefully placed in the eluent in the chamber. This makes sure that the solvent level does not go above the origin line. The watch glass goes back over the beaker.
8. **Elution and Visualization:** When the solvent front gets about 1 cm from the top edge of the plate, take the plate off and use a pencil to mark the highest point of the solvent front. Then, the plate is left to dry. It can see the separated spots, which are very colorful curcuminoids. For each visible spot, the retention factor (Rf) value is found. To make the spots easier to see, dip the dried TLC plate in a 0.5% w/v boric acid solution in a 1:1 ethanol:water mixture. This is because compounds react with boric acid to make brighter orange products.

**Precautions:**

- Turmeric can leave permanent stains on clothes, surfaces, and skin, so it's important to wear gloves and a lab coat.

- To keep skin oils from getting on TLC plates, you should only touch the edges of the plates. Skin oils can change the way chromatographic separation works.
- All work with solvents should be done in a fume hood so that solvent vapors don't get into the air. Also, silica dust can damage the lungs if breathed in, so be careful.

**Result:** Curcumin from *Curcuma longa* Rhizomes was isolated.

## EXPERIMENT No: 04

**Object:** Isolation of Caffeine from Tea Leaves.

**Requirements:**

**Reagents:**

- Tea leaves
- Calcium carbonate
- Water
- Methylene chloride
- Anhydrous magnesium sulfate
- Acetone
- Petroleum ether
- For TLC: Pure caffeine standard, 50% CH3OH/H2O

**Equipment:**

- 600 mL beaker
- Hot plate
- Buchner funnel
- Filter paper
- 500 mL separatory funnel
- Powder funnel
- Cotton plug
- Roto-evaporator
- 100-mL round-bottom flask
- 50 mL Erlenmeyer flask
- Boiling stick
- Steam bath
- Small Hirsch funnel
- Sealed vial
- Analytical balance
- TLC plate
- UV light

**Theory**:

Separating caffeine from tea leaves is a great way to show how liquid-liquid extraction and recrystallization work. These are important steps in natural product chemistry. Caffeine is a small part of tea leaves, but it is an important bioactive compound.

**Procedure:**

1. **Boiling Tea Leaves:** In a 600 mL beaker, 15 g of tea leaves, 5 g of calcium carbonate powder, and 200 mL of water are combined. The mixture is then boiled on a hot plate for 20 minutes, with intermittent stirring. The inclusion of calcium carbonate is a strategic step; it aids in precipitating water-soluble impurities such as tannins and

gallic acid as insoluble calcium salts, thereby preventing their co-extraction with caffeine.

2. **Hot Filtration:** The solution is allowed to cool slightly but is filtered while still warm through a Buchner funnel using a fast filter paper. It is important to note that hot solutions are typically not vacuum filtered, but this is an exception for caffeine extraction due to its solubility profile. The tea leaves are rinsed twice with 50 mL portions of water, and as much filtrate as possible is carefully pressed out, as caffeine is primarily in the aqueous layer.
3. **Liquid-Liquid Extraction (Methylene Chloride):** The filtrate is cooled to room temperature and transferred to a 500 mL separatory funnel. A 35 mL aliquot of methylene chloride is added for the first extraction. The separatory funnel is vigorously shaken, with frequent venting to relieve pressure buildup, to extract caffeine into the organic layer. This extraction is repeated two more times with fresh 35 mL aliquots of methylene chloride to maximize caffeine recovery, as caffeine is quite soluble in methylene chloride.
4. **Drying Organic Layer:** The combined methylene chloride extracts are collected. If an emulsion forms, the methylene chloride layer is slowly drained through a small amount of anhydrous magnesium sulfate placed in a powder funnel with a loose cotton plug; this effectively breaks the emulsion. Additional anhydrous magnesium sulfate is added if further drying of the organic layer is required.
5. **Evaporation:** The dried methylene chloride solution is transferred to a tared 100-mL round-bottom flask. The methylene chloride is then removed by stripping to dryness using a roto-evaporator, a process that typically takes less than 5 minutes. A small amount of greenish residue, representing crude caffeine, will remain.
6. **Recrystallization:** The crude caffeine is dissolved in 5-8 mL of hot acetone in a 50 mL Erlenmeyer flask. Petroleum ether is added dropwise until the "cloud point" is reached, indicating that caffeine is beginning to precipitate due to reduced solubility in the mixed solvent system. The solution is then cooled to promote crystallization. If no precipitate forms, excess acetone is carefully boiled off using a boiling stick, and more petroleum ether is added until crystallization is initiated.
7. **Collection & Drying:** The recrystallized caffeine is collected by suction filtration

using a small Hirsch funnel, with cold petroleum ether serving as a rinse solvent. A second crop of caffeine may form in the filtrate as the solvent evaporates and can be collected similarly, but it should be kept separate from the first crop. The collected crystals are then air-dried.

8. **TLC Analysis (for Purity Monitoring):** To monitor the purity and progress of the extraction, samples of crude and recrystallized caffeine, alongside a pure caffeine standard, are spotted onto a TLC plate. The plate is developed with a 50% CH3OH/H2O solvent system, and spots are visualized under UV light to determine their Rf values.

**Precautions:**

- Students are mandated to wear goggles and gloves for this experiment.
- Proper waste disposal protocols for potassium carbonate, aqueous solutions, and organic solutions must be followed.
- Methylene chloride is a volatile organic solvent, necessitating work in a well-ventilated area or fume hood.
- Pressure buildup in the separatory funnel must be relieved frequently during shaking.

**Result:** Caffeine from Tea Leaves was isolated.

## EXPERIMENT No: 05

**Object:** Isolation of Ammonium Glycyrrhizinate from Liquorice.

**Requirement:**

**Reagents:**

- Liquorice root powder
- Ethanol
- Water
- Methanol
- Acetic acid (for HPLC mobile phase)
- Glycyrrhizic acid (mono-ammonium salt hydrate) standard (for calibration)

**Equipment:**

- Oven (for drying liquorice roots)
- Crusher (for powdering liquorice roots)
- Stirring apparatus (for dipping extraction)
- Hydrothermal extractor (if using the hydrothermal method)
- HPLC system: solvent delivery pump, UV detector, data system, injection valve, column
- Disposable syringe filter unit
- Decompressing pump

**Theory:** The extraction of ammonium glycyrrhizinate (mono ammonium glycyrrhizate) from liquorice root (Glycyrrhiza glabra) is a crucial process for acquiring this bioactive compound recognized for its therapeutic attributes. This section explains both advanced and more traditional ways to extract substances on a laboratory scale. It then talks about high-performance liquid chromatography (HPLC) for separation and determination.

**Procedure**

1. **Sample Preparation:** Liquorice root powder serves as the starting material for extraction.
2. **Hydrothermal Extraction (Optimal Parameters):** For optimal extraction of monoammonium glycyrrhizate, hydrothermal technology is employed under specific conditions: 200°C, a duration of 30.29 minutes, and a pressure of 0.5 MPa. This method is recognized for its sustainability, as it eliminates the need for harmful organic solvents, thereby reducing environmental impact and health risks.
3. **Alternative Extraction (Ethanol/Water Dipping):** A more accessible laboratory-scale approach involves using an ethanol/water mixture (30:70, v/v) as the extraction solvent. The liquorice powder is mixed and stirred with the solvent, followed by a 60-minute dipping period at 50°C. While ultrasonic extraction is another option, it has been noted to yield lower amounts of the target compounds and requires more energy.
4. **Separation/Determination (HPLC):** The obtained extracts are further separated and quantified using reversed-phase high-performance liquid chromatography (RP-HPLC).

**Mobile Phase:** A mixture of methanol/water (70:30, v/v) containing 1% acetic acid is used as the mobile phase.

**Column:** A C18 column (5μm particle size, 150×4.6 mm dimensions) is typically employed.

**Detection:** A UV detector is used to monitor the eluting compounds.

**Sample Preparation for HPLC:** Prior to injection into the HPLC system, the extract is filtered through a 0.2 μm disposable syringe filter unit to remove any particulate matter that could interfere with the analysis or damage the column.

**Precautions:**

General laboratory safety protocols for handling solvents and operating high-pressure and high-temperature equipment must be strictly observed.

**Result:** Ammonium Glycyrrhizinate from Liquorice was isolated.

## EXPERIMENT No: 06

**Object:** Isolation of Piperine from *Piper longum.*

**Requirement:**

**Reagents:**

- Black pepper (ground)
- 95% ethanol
- 10% alcoholic KOH

**Equipments:**

- Soxhlet extractor (with thimble and round-bottomed flask)
- Whatman filter paper
- Distillation/evaporation equipment (e.g., rotary evaporator)
- Glassware (beakers, measuring cylinders, funnels)
- pH indicator strips (optional for process monitoring)
- Separatory funnel (for general extraction, though not explicitly for this specific Soxhlet protocol).

**Theory:** Separating piperine, an alkaloid that gives black pepper (Piper nigrum or Piper longum) its strong smell, is a useful process that shows how Soxhlet extraction and recrystallization work. Piperine is also known for its possible health benefits.

**Procedure (Soxhlet Extraction & Recrystallization):**

1. **Grinding:** A quantity of 10 g of black pepper is ground to a coarse powder. This increases the surface area, facilitating a more efficient extraction process.
2. **Soxhlet Extraction:** The ground pepper is carefully placed into a thimble (a porous bag) within a Soxhlet extraction apparatus. In the round-bottomed flask below, 200 mL of 95% ethanol is added. The extraction is allowed to proceed for 3 hours. During this process, the ethanol continuously cycles through heating, evaporation, condensation over the pepper, and siphoning back to the flask, thereby dissolving and concentrating the piperine from the plant material.

3. **Concentration:** After extraction, the solution is allowed to cool. It is then filtered through Whatman filter paper. The solution is subsequently concentrated, typically by evaporation, to remove most of the ethanol, reducing the volume to approximately 5 mL.
4. **Alkaline Treatment:** To the concentrated residue, 10 mL of 10% alcoholic KOH is added, and the mixture is allowed to stand for 1 hour. This step is crucial for purification, as the strong base (KOH) can precipitate acidic impurities or hydrolyze co-extracted compounds that are soluble in ethanol but insoluble under alkaline conditions, thereby enhancing the purity of the target alkaloid.
5. **Decantation & Crystallization:** The solution is carefully decanted from any insoluble residue that may have formed. The alcoholic solution is then left undisturbed overnight, or for 24–48 hours, to allow long yellow needles of piperine to crystallize and deposit.
6. **Collection & Washing:** The yellow needle-like crystals of piperine are collected, typically by filtration. They are then washed with a minimum volume of 95% ethanol to remove any adhering impurities.
7. **Drying & Characterization:** The collected crystals are allowed to air dry. Their weight is determined, and the melting point is measured to assess purity. Further purification, if necessary, can be achieved through additional recrystallization steps. Analytical techniques such as Thin Layer Chromatography (TLC) or spectroscopy can be employed to confirm the purity and identity of the isolated piperine.

**Precautions:**

- Strict adherence to safety guidelines is imperative when working with solvents.
- Extraction procedures should always be conducted in a well-ventilated area, preferably a fume hood, and appropriate protective equipment (e.g., gloves, lab coat, eye protection) must be worn.
- Ethanol is a flammable solvent and should be handled with care, away from ignition sources.

**Result:** Isolation of Piperine from Piper longum was done.

# EXPERIMENT No: 07

**Object:** Study of Methods of Extraction.

**Requirements:**

- General containers (test tubes, beakers, flasks)
- Heating apparatus (water baths, ovens, hot plates)
- Filtration apparatus (funnels, filter paper)
- Specialized equipment for continuous extraction (Soxhlet extractor, percolator)
- Advanced systems (microwave extractor, ultrasonic extractor).

**Theory:** Extraction is the foundational and most critical step in natural product research. Its primary objective is to selectively separate bioactive substances from their inactive or inert components within the plant matrix, utilizing appropriate solvents and techniques. A comprehensive understanding of various extraction methods is indispensable for optimizing the yield, purity, and stability of plant-derived compounds, which directly impacts their suitability for further research or pharmaceutical development.

**Principles and Procedures:**

1. **Maceration:**

This traditional method involves soaking coarsely powdered plant material in a solvent (menstruum) within a closed container for a minimum of three days. Periodic stirring or shaking ensures thorough solvent penetration and dissolution of active constituents. The resulting extract (micelle) is then separated from the insoluble residue (marc) by filtration or decantation, followed by solvent evaporation.

***Advantage:*** Simple, convenient, and suitable for thermolabile (heat-sensitive) plant materials.

2. **Infusion:** Similar to maceration, this process involves soaking finely powdered drug material in hot or cold solvent for a short duration. The solvent-to-sample ratio typically ranges from 4:1 to 16:1.

***Advantage:*** Effective for readily soluble bioactive constituents and ideal for preparing fresh extracts for immediate use.

3. **Digestion:** This method is a variation of maceration that incorporates moderate heat (approximately 50°C) during the extraction process. The applied heat reduces the viscosity of the extraction solvent, thereby enhancing the removal of secondary metabolites.

***Advantage:*** Suitable for readily soluble plant materials.

4.**Decoction:** This method involves continuous hot extraction using a specified volume of water as a solvent for dried, powdered plant material, typically for about 15 minutes. The solvent-to-crude drug ratio is usually 4:1 or 16:1.

o ***Advantage:*** Employed for the extraction of water-soluble and heat-stable plant materials.

5.**Percolation:** In this process, moistened, finely powdered plant material is packed into a percolator, a narrow-cone-shaped glass vessel. The solvent is poured from the top and allowed to slowly drip through the material due to gravitational force. Continuous addition of solvent ensures complete extraction until the desired volume is collected. The extract is then filtered and decanted.

***Advantage:*** Efficient for extracting large amounts of drug using relatively smaller solvent volumes.

6.**Soxhlet Extraction (Continuous Hot Extraction):** Dried, finely powdered plant material is placed in a porous thimble within a Soxhlet apparatus. The solvent in a bottom flask is heated, evaporates, condenses over the material, and siphons back to the flask, continuously extracting the drug. This cycle repeats until the extraction is complete, typically indicated when the solvent returning from the extraction chamber leaves no residue.

***Advantage:*** Enables the extraction of large amounts of drug with less solvent, eliminates the need for filtration, and is applicable to heat-stable plant materials.

***Disadvantage:*** Not suitable for thermolabile materials, and regular shaking is not possible.

7. **Microwave-Assisted Extraction (MAE):** This technique utilizes electromagnetic radiation (microwaves) to heat the solvent and plant matrix, thereby facilitating solvent

penetration and extraction. Microwaves applied at frequencies between 300 MHz and 300 GHz (wavelengths between 1 cm and 1 m) are commonly used, with 2450 Hz yielding energy between 600 and 700 W.

***Advantage:*** Minimizes solvent consumption and extraction time, and increases yield.

***Disadvantage:*** Primarily suitable for phenolic compounds and flavonoids; tannins and anthocyanins may degrade due to high temperatures; not favorable for nonpolar solvents.

8. **Ultrasound-Assisted Extraction (UAE):** This method applies high-frequency sound energy (>20 KHz) to disrupt plant cell walls, increasing the surface area of the drug for solvent penetration and facilitating the release of secondary metabolites.

   ***Advantage:*** Applicable to small samples, reduces extraction time and solvent volume, and maximizes yield.

   ***Disadvantage:*** Can be difficult to reproduce, and high energy may lead to the degradation of phytochemicals by producing free radicals.

**Precautions:**

- An ideal solvent for extraction should be nontoxic and nonflammable.
- Certain solvents, such as chloroform, are noted for their sedative and carcinogenic properties, while alcohol is flammable and volatile.
- Microwave-assisted and ultrasound-assisted extraction methods can involve high temperatures and energy, posing potential risks.
- General laboratory safety protocols, including proper ventilation, the use of appropriate personal protective equipment (PPE), and careful handling of all chemicals and heated equipment, are paramount for all extraction procedures.

**Result:** Different methods of Extraction was studied.

# EXPERIMENT No: 08

**Object:** Phytochemical Screening of Selected Plants.

**Requirements:**

**Reagents:**

Plant extract, 1% HCl, Mayer-Wagner reagent (2.5 gm iodine in 12.5 gm KI2 with 250 mL distilled water), 0.1% Ferric chloride, Distilled water, Ethanol, Concentrated HCl, Magnesium ribbon, NaOH, Chloroform, Sulfuric acid, FeCl3, K2Fe(CN)6, Specific reagents for Dragendorff's, Hager's, and Wagner's tests for alkaloids.

**Equipments:**

Beakers, Conical flasks, Measuring cylinders, Glass funnels, Glass stirrer, Test tubes, Bunsen burner, Weighing balance (top mettler and analytical), Water bath (thermostat), Mortar and pestle, Capillary tubes.

**Theory:**

Preliminary phytochemical screening serves as the initial and fundamental phase in the extensive phytochemical analysis of botanical specimens. This qualitative evaluation seeks to ascertain the existence or non-existence of principal categories of secondary metabolites, including alkaloids, flavonoids, phenols, saponins, steroids, tannins, terpenoids, and glycosides, in plant extracts. The information obtained from this screening is essential for comprehending the potential therapeutic attributes of plants and for directing more focused and resource-intensive quantitative analyses and drug discovery initiatives.

**Procedure:**

1) **Extract Preparation:** Plant extracts are typically prepared by dissolving the plant material in a suitable solvent, such as water or ethanol.
2) **Specific Tests:** A series of specific chemical tests are then performed for each class of phytochemical, with observations made for characteristic color changes or the formation of precipitates.

**Specific Tests and Observations:**

i. **Alkaloids:**

- **Mayer-Wagner Test:** The plant extract is dissolved in 100 mL of water and filtered. A 2 mL aliquot of the filtrate is heated in steam with three drops of 1% HCl. Subsequently, 1 mL of the heated mixture is combined with 6 mL of Mayer-Wagner reagent (prepared by dissolving 2.5 gm of iodine in 12.5 gm of KI2 with 250 mL of distilled water).

  ***Observation:*** The formation of a cream or brown-red colored precipitate indicates the presence of alkaloids.

  **Other Tests:** Additional qualitative tests for alkaloids include Dragendorff's test (producing an orange-red precipitate), Hager's test (yielding a creamy white precipitate), and Wagner's test (resulting in a reddish precipitate).

ii. **Tannins:** Approximately 200 mg of the plant extract is boiled with 10 mL of distilled water. To this, 0.1% Ferric chloride solution is added.

***Observation:*** A blue-black coloration confirms the presence of tannins.

iii. **Saponins:** About 0.5 mL of the extract is combined with 5 mL of distilled water and agitated vigorously.

***Observation:*** The formation of persistent foam indicates the presence of saponins.

iv. **Flavonoids:** A 200 mg portion of the plant extract is mixed with 10 mL of ethanol and filtered. Two mL of the filtrate is then mixed with concentrated HCl and a piece of magnesium ribbon.

***Observation:*** The appearance of a pink or red color signifies the presence of flavonoids.

v. **Glycosides:** To 0.5 mL of crude extract, 1 mL of distilled water and NaOH are added.

***Observation:*** The formation of a yellowish color suggests the presence of glycosides.

vi. **Steroids:** Approximately 1 mL of the crude extract is combined with 10 mL of chloroform and 10 mL of sulfuric acid.

***Observation:*** The formation of a distinct bilayer, with a red top layer and a greenish bottom layer, indicates the presence of steroids.

vii. **Terpenoids:** A 0.5 mL aliquot of crude extract is mixed with 2 mL of chloroform and 3 mL of sulfuric acid.

***Observation:*** The development of a reddish-brown color confirms the presence of terpenoids.

viii. **Phenols:** About 1 mL of the extract is combined with three drops of $FeCl_3$ and 1 mL of $K_2Fe(CN)_6$.

***Observation:*** The formation of greenish-blue coloration confirms the presence of phenols.

**Precautions:**

Wear appropriate personal protective equipment (PPE), such as lab coats, gloves, and eye protection. When handling volatile or corrosive chemicals (e.g., concentrated HCl, sulfuric acid, chloroform), work should be done in a fume hood. Proper disposal of all chemical waste is also crucial.

**Result:** Phytochemical Screening of Selected Plants was done.

## EXPERIMENT No: 09

**Object:** Chromatographic and spectrophotometric analysis of natural products using Thin Layer Chromatography (TLC) of plant extracts.

**Requirements:**

**Reagents:**

- Plant extracts
- Solvents for extraction and concentration (e.g., methanol, ethanol, ethyl ether)
- Cleaning solvent (e.g., ethyl acetate-methanol 2:1 v/v)
- Mobile phase (e.g., ethyl acetate-methanol 4:1 v/v, or 70:30 cyclohexane:isopropanol for curcuminoids)
- Standards of known compounds
- For bioautography: Microbial suspensions, agar, tetrazolium red

**Equipments:**

- TLC plates (silica gel, aluminum/plastic-backed)
- Scissors
- Fume hood
- TLC developing chambers (glass beakers/jars with lids)
- Filter paper
- Microliter syringe/capillary micropipettes
- Forceps/tongs
- UV lamp (254 nm/365 nm)
- Drying oven

**Theory:** Thin Layer Chromatography (TLC) is a simple, quick, and cheap way to separate and identify the different parts of a mixture. It plays a big role in the quality control, authentication, and standardization of herbal medicines because it makes it easy to quickly identify and fingerprint plant-based compounds.

The basic idea behind TLC is that compounds interact differently with two phases: a stationary phase and a mobile phase. In most cases, the stationary phase is a thin layer of solid absorbent (like silica gel) on top of an inert base (like glass, aluminum foil, or plastic that doesn't dissolve). The mobile phase is a solvent or a mixture of solvents that moves up the plate by capillary action. As the mobile phase moves, compounds separate based on their size, charge, solubility, or polarity. In "normal phase" TLC, a polar stationary phase is used with a less polar mobile phase. This makes more polar molecules stick to the stationary phase better, which slows down their movement and lowers their Retention factor (Rf) values.

**Procedure:**

1. **Extract Preparation:** Plant extracts must be concentrated to allow for application to TLC plates in a minimal volume. Extracts are dissolved in an appropriate organic solvent, such as methanol, to create a concentrated solution rather than a turbid suspension.
2. **Plate Preparation:** TLC plates (typically aluminum- or plastic-backed silica gel) are cleaned by developing them in a polar, neutral solvent (e.g., ethyl acetate-methanol 2:1 v/v) to remove any adsorbed contaminants from the development zone. The plates are then dried in a fume hood, followed by further drying in an oven (e.g., 100°C for 10-15 minutes) to eliminate residual moisture that could affect compound migration.
3. **Developing Chamber Preparation:** A piece of filter paper is cut to serve as a wick inside the TLC developing chamber. The mobile phase solvents (e.g., ethyl acetate-methanol 4:1 v/v) are mixed and poured into the chamber. The chamber is then covered and allowed to saturate with solvent vapors, which improves reproducibility of separations.
4. **Sample Loading:** A horizontal pencil line is lightly marked as the origin, approximately 1 cm from the bottom edge of the TLC plate. Concentrated samples and standards are then loaded as narrow bands onto this line using a microliter syringe or capillary micropipettes. The loaded bands are allowed to dry. If a greater sample concentration is required, "overspotting" (repeated application on the same spot) can be performed.
5. **Development:** The TLC plate(s) are carefully placed into the saturated chamber using forceps or tongs, ensuring that the solvent level remains below the origin line and that the plates do not touch the wick. The chamber is covered, and the plate is allowed to develop until the solvent front reaches approximately 1 cm from the top edge.
6. **Visualization:** After development, the plate is removed, and the solvent front is immediately marked with a pencil. The plate is then dried in a fume hood. Separated bands are visualized under visible light or ultraviolet (UV) light (typically at 254 nm

and 365 nm) and delineated with a pencil.

7. **Rf Calculation:** The Retention factor (Rf) value for each spot is calculated using the formula: Rf = (distance traveled by compound) / (distance traveled by solvent front). The Rf value is a characteristic property of a compound in a specific solvent system at a particular temperature.
8. **Bioautography (Optional for Antimicrobial Activity):** For screening antimicrobial compounds, the chromatograms can be exposed to microbial suspensions (e.g., fungi or bacteria in agar). After allowing time for microbial growth in a humid environment, zones of inhibition are visualized by staining the agar plates with tetrazolium red.

**Precautions:**

- All work involving solvents and silica dust should be performed in a fume hood to prevent inhalation.
- Gloves must be worn when handling TLC plates to prevent contamination from skin oils.
- It is important to be aware that silica can cause lung damage if inhaled.
- When performing bioautography, strict sterile techniques are essential to prevent microbial contamination.

**Result:** Chromatographic and spectrophotometric analysis of natural products using Thin Layer Chromatography (TLC) of plant extracts was done.

# EXPERIMENT No: 10

**Object:** Fingerprinting of selected medicinal plant extracts using High-Performance Thin-Layer Chromatography (HPTLC).

**Requirements:**

HPTLC plates, automatic TLC sampler, automatic developing chamber , CAMAG HP-TLC Visualisation Analyser system

**Theory:**

High-Performance Thin-Layer Chromatography (HPTLC) is a big step forward from regular TLC because it has better resolution, higher detection sensitivity, and better in situ quantification. This makes HPTLC a powerful and advanced tool for both qualitative and quantitative analysis of plants and herbal remedies. It is widely used for quality control, checking the authenticity of herbal drugs, and doing full fingerprint analysis. Principles: HPTLC uses smaller plates that are covered in very fine, evenly sized particles of adsorbents. These are usually silica gel, but they can also be alumina or cellulose. This optimized stationary phase makes chromatography work better by spreading the bands out more evenly and giving them better resolution. The method makes a "fingerprint," which is a unique sequence of peaks or zones that is specific to the chemical parts of the extract. This serves as a unique identifier for the plant material.

**Procedure (General for HPTLC Fingerprinting):**

1. **Sample Preparation:** The medicinal plant material (e.g., Ashwagandha, Tulsi, Bael, Amla, Ginger, Aloe, Vidang, Senna, Lawsonia) is extracted using appropriate solvents. The extraction protocol typically involves grinding the plant material, followed by sonication, and successive extraction with solvents of increasing polarity (e.g., n-hexane, ethyl acetate, methanol).
2. **Plate Preparation:** HPTLC plates (e.g., silica gel, 10x10 cm or 10x20 cm) are used. Prior to use, plates are inspected for any damage or impurities and prewashed to enhance reproducibility.
3. **Sample Application:** Samples and reference standards are applied precisely onto the

HPTLC plate using high-tech equipment designed for accurate sample application.

4. **Chromatogram Development:** The chromatogram is developed using a standardized and reproducible method. Mobile phases are carefully selected based on the specific class of compounds being analyzed (e.g., chloroform-methanol for alkaloids, or a mixture of formic acid, water, methyl ethyl ketone, and ethyl acetate for flavonoids). A modern approach involves using three complementary developing solvents (CDS) to ensure effective separation of all components.
5. **Derivatization/Visualization:** After development, specific spray reagents (derivatization reagents) are applied to the plate to visualize different compound classes. Examples include Dragendorff's reagent for alkaloids, NP and PEG reagents for flavonoids, Fast blue salt B for polyphenols, and 10% sulfuric acid for terpenoids. Heat may be applied to facilitate the reaction. Visualization is performed under visible light or UV light (typically at 365 nm).
6. **Documentation & Evaluation:** The developed chromatograms are documented and evaluated using software-controlled systems, such as the CAMAG HP-TLC Visualisation Analyser system. This system provides advanced image acquisition, multi-spectral detection, automated documentation, and data integration capabilities for quantitative evaluations and digital fingerprinting.

**Table:** HPTLC Conditions for Phytochemical Fingerprinting

| Compound Class | Mobile Phase Examples | Spray Reagent | Heat | Visible Light Observation | UV (365 nm) Observation |
|---|---|---|---|---|---|
| **Alkaloids** | Chloroform-met hanol (30:13, v/v) | Dragendorff's reagent | RT for 10 min | Yellow | Dark blue, dark violet |
| **Flavonoids** | Formic acid - water - methyl ethyl ketone - ethyl acetate (1:1:3:5, v/v/v/v) | NP and PEG | 100°C for 3 min | Yellow, red | Yellow, green |

| Polyphenols | Chloroform - ethyl acetate - methanol – water (15:50:22:10, v/v/v/v) | Fast blue salt B | RT for max 10 min | Purple, orange, brown | Dark violet |
|---|---|---|---|---|---|
| **Terpenoids** | Toluene - ethyl acetate - methanol - formic acid - acetic acid (100:15:10:2:1, v/v/v/v/v) | 10% sulfuric acid (v/v) in methanol | 100°C for 3 min | Violet, purple | Violet, purple |

**Result:**

# EXPERIMENT No: 11

**Object:** Analysis of Pharmacopoeial compounds of natural origin and their formulations by UV-Visible Spectrophotometer.

**Requirements:**

**Reagents:** Sample, Suitable solvents , Standards of the target compound.

**Equipment:** UV-Vis spectrophotometer, Cuvettes.

**Principle:** UV-Vis spectrophotometry works by measuring how much ultraviolet and visible light a sample absorbs. This is the range of energy that most molecules and ions with chromophores absorb. This makes electrons move to higher energy molecular orbitals. The Beer-Lambert law is the most important rule for quantitative analysis in UV-Vis spectroscopy. It says that the absorbance of a solution is directly related to the concentration of the absorbing species in the solution and the path length of the light through the sample.

**Procedure (General for Quantitative Analysis):**

1. **Sample Preparation:** The sample, whether a pharmacopoeial compound or an herbal formulation, is dissolved in a suitable solvent. Common choices include water for water-soluble compounds or ethanol for organic-soluble compounds. It is important to note that solvent polarity and pH can influence the absorption spectrum of an organic compound. The prepared solution in the cuvette should be transparent and non-absorbing in the target wavelength range.
2. **Blank Measurement:** A cuvette containing only the solvent (the blank) is placed in the spectrophotometer. A light beam is passed through it, and the intensity of the transmitted light is measured across different wavelengths. This measurement is recorded as the blank, serving as a reference for subsequent sample determinations.
3. **Sample Measurement:** The sample, dissolved in the same solvent, is placed in a cuvette. A light beam is passed through the sample, and the light is partially absorbed by the sample molecules in the solution.
4. **Absorbance Calculation:** The intensity of the light transmitted through the sample is measured. The change in light intensity at different wavelengths is calculated by dividing

the transmitted intensity of the sample solution by the corresponding values obtained from the blank. This ratio is then used to calculate absorbance ($A = -\log(T)$), which is typically plotted against wavelength to generate the UV-Vis spectrum.

5. **Quantitative Determination (using Beer-Lambert Law):**

- The spectrum of the target compound shows its maximum absorption wavelength ($\lambda$max).
- To make a calibration curve, you measure the absorbance of several known concentrations of a pure standard compound at its $\lambda$max. You make a graph of absorbance against concentration.
- The unknown sample's absorbance is measured at the same $\lambda$max. If you know the extinction coefficient ($\varepsilon$) and path length (d), you can then use the established calibration curve or the Beer-Lambert law ($A = \varepsilon * c * d$) to find the concentration of the unknown sample.
- For the best results and to follow the Beer-Lambert Law, absorbance readings should be in the instrument's linear range, which is usually between 0.01 and 2.5 absorbance units.

**Result:** Pharmacopoeial compounds of natural origin and their formulations by UV-Visible Spectrophotometer were analysed.

# EXPERIMENT No: 12

**Object:** Analysis of recorded spectra of simple phytoconstituents.

**Requirement:** UV-Vis spectrophotometer

**Principle:** The usefulness of UV-Vis spectroscopy in structural analysis comes from the fact that different functional groups and conjugated systems in organic molecules absorb light at specific wavelengths in the UV or visible parts of the electromagnetic spectrum. The specific position and profile (shape and intensity) of these absorption peaks act as a unique fingerprint for certain compounds.

**Procedure:**

1. **Obtain Spectrum:** The UV-Vis spectrum of the phytoconstituent is acquired, either directly from a spectrophotometer or from a reliable spectral database.
2. **Identify Absorption Peaks:** The maximum absorption wavelengths ($\lambda max$) are identified, and the shape and intensity of these peaks are carefully observed.
3. **Correlate with Functional Groups:** The observed wavelengths of absorption peaks are correlated with known chromophores and functional groups (e.g., carbonyl groups (C=O), conjugated double bonds) that are characteristic of organic molecules.
4. **Assess Purity:** The spectrum is analyzed for any unexpected peaks or deviations from the known spectrum of a pure standard compound. Such anomalies can indicate the presence of impurities or degradation products.
5. **Influence of Environment:** It is important to consider how external factors, such as solvent polarity and pH, can influence the absorption spectrum. These factors can lead to observable shifts in absorption maxima and changes in molar extinction coefficients.
   - **Precautions:** General laboratory safety practices should be followed when handling samples and solvents.

**Result:**

# EXPERIMENT No: 13

**Object:** Demonstration of High-Performance Liquid Chromatography (HPLC) with natural product extracts.

**Requirements:**

HPLC system, Syringe filters, Glassware for sample and mobile phase preparation

**Principle:** HPLC works by separating parts of a mixture based on how their chemical properties differ from one another. This is done by pushing a liquid mobile phase through a column filled with a stationary phase at a high pressure. Because the compounds react differently with the stationary and mobile phases, they come out of the column at different times, which separates them. People often use a UV-Vis spectrophotometer as an HPLC detector. It measures how much light eluting compounds absorb at certain wavelengths.

Procedure:

1. **Sample Preparation:** A concentrated solution of the natural product extract is prepared in a suitable solvent. Prior to injection, the sample is filtered through a syringe filter (e.g., 0.2 µm pore size) to remove any particulate matter that could damage the column or interfere with the analysis.
2. **Mobile Phase Preparation:** The mobile phase, a mixture of solvents (e.g., methanol/water containing 1% acetic acid for glycyrrhizic acid analysis), is prepared. It is crucial to degas the mobile phase to prevent air bubbles from interfering with the pump and detector.
3. **System Setup:** The HPLC system is assembled, comprising a solvent delivery pump, an injector, a chromatographic column (e.g., a C18 reversed-phase column), and a detector (e.g., a UV detector).
4. **Method Development/Selection:** Appropriate chromatographic conditions are selected or developed. These include parameters such as flow rate, column temperature, and detection wavelength, which are optimized based on the chemical properties of the target compounds.
5. **Injection:** A precise volume of the prepared sample is injected into the HPLC system.

6. **Separation & Detection:** As the sample passes through the column, its components are separated and then detected as they elute, generating a chromatogram (a plot of detector response versus time).
7. **Analysis:** The chromatogram is analyzed to identify and quantify compounds based on their characteristic retention times and peak areas, which are compared against those of known standards.

**Result:**

High-Performance Liquid Chromatography (HPLC) with natural product extracts was demonstrated.

## EXPERIMENT No: 14

**Object:** Quantitative Estimation of Aldehyde/Phenolic Content in Herbal Raw Materials.

**Requirements:**

**For Phenolic Content**

**Reagents:** Plant extract, Folin- Ciocalteu reagent, Na2CO3 solution, Gallic acid standard

**Equipment**: Spectrophotometer (UV-Vis), Cuvettes, test tubes, pipettes

**For Aldehyde Content**

**Reagents:** Purified cotton cellulose or hydro celluloses, Hydrochloric acid, 0.2M sodium carbonate

**Equipment:** Erlenmeyer flask, Thermostat, Pipettes, Burette

**Theory:** Quantitative estimation of aldehyde or total phenolic content (TPC) in herbal raw materials is crucial for various applications, including assessing degradation in cellulosic materials (for aldehyde content) and correlating TPC with antioxidant activity in plant extracts.

**Procedure (Phenolic Content - Folin-Ciocalteu Method):**

1. **Sample Preparation:** The plant extract is prepared, typically dissolved in water or ethanol.

   **Reaction:** The Folin-Ciocalteu (FC) assay involves the reaction of phenolic compounds with the Folin-Ciocalteu reagent, which oxidizes the phenolics. This redox reaction results in the formation of a blue-colored reduced FC reagent, which is then measured spectrophotometrically.

2. **pH Optimization:** The traditional FC assay, often performed with a 7.50% aqueous Na2CO3 solution at pH 10.8, can lead to a significant overestimation of TPC due to interference from reducing sugars. To mitigate this, an optimized pH of 7.9, achieved by using a 0.75% aqueous Na2CO3 solution, is employed. This condition minimizes sugar interference while still allowing for the accurate quantification of most phenolic compounds. This highlights that even standardized quantitative methods require

careful optimization when applied to complex natural products to ensure accuracy and prevent overestimation. The presence of other compounds, like sugars, can significantly skew results, necessitating method validation and refinement.

3. **Measurement:** The absorbance of the reaction mixture is measured at 760 nm. The intensity of the blue color observed is directly proportional to the sample's phenolics content.
4. **Standard Curve:** A standard curve is prepared by measuring the absorbance of known concentrations of a reference phenolic compound (e.g., gallic acid equivalents, GAE).
5. **Calculation:** The TPC of the sample is determined by comparing its measured absorbance to the established standard curve.

**Procedure (Aldehyde Content - Iodine Titration):**

1. **Sample Preparation:** For the estimation of aldehyde content in cellulosic materials, purified cotton cellulose can be initially dewaxed by extraction with hot alcohol for 24 hours and further purified by boiling with a 1% sodium hydroxide solution for 8 hours. Hydrocelluloses, if used, are prepared by steeping samples of purified cotton in hydrochloric acid solutions (0.5 to 5.0 N) for 24 hours at 21°C.
2. **Titration Setup:** A 100 mL aliquot of a buffer solution (e.g., approximately pH 10.6, prepared by mixing 15 parts of 0.2M sodium carbonate and 1 part of 0.2M sodium bicarbonate) is pipetted into a 500-mL glass-stoppered Erlenmeyer flask and cooled to 0°C. Subsequently, 25 mL of a 0.0500 N iodine solution (containing 40 g of potassium iodide per liter), also pre-cooled to 0°C, is added.
3. **Sample Introduction:** The sample to be titrated (e.g., 0.05 g of glucose or approximately 1 g of cotton) is immediately introduced into the flask.
4. **Reaction & Titration:** The reaction is allowed to proceed. The mixture is then titrated with thiosulfate. Near the endpoint, the solution becomes nearly colorless, although the fiber may retain a brown color if cotton is used. At this point, thiosulfate addition is paused, and the mixture is vigorously shaken (with frequent release of the stopper to vent CO2) to ensure complete reaction.
5. **Correction:** A correction is applied for any slow side reactions that may consume iodine over time. The iodine consumed in this manner converts aldehyde groups to carboxyl groups, a conversion that can be independently verified by estimating the

carboxyl groups formed via titration with silver o-nitrophenolate.

**Precautions:**

- Folin-Ciocalteu reagent contains phosphotungstate-phosphomolybdate, which can be corrosive and should be handled with care.
- Iodine solutions and the strong acids and bases used in aldehyde estimation necessitate the use of appropriate personal protective equipment (PPE) and work within a fume hood.
- Proper disposal of all chemical waste is essential.

**Result:** Quantitative Estimation of Aldehyde/Phenolic Content in Herbal Raw Materials was done.

# EXPERIMENT No: 15

**Object:** Estimation of Alkaloid Content in Herbal Raw Materials.

**Requirements:**

**Reagents:** Plant material, Methanol, Dragendorff's reagent, Bromocresol green, 2N NaOH, Distilled water, Sodium phosphate, Citric acid, Atropine standard.

**Equipment:** Soxhlet apparatus, Rotary evaporator, Volumetric flasks, Beakers, Pipettes, Test tubes, Digital balance, Colorimeter or UV-Spectrophotometer, Heating mantle

**Principles:**

Alkaloids can be extracted from plant material using various techniques, such as Soxhlet extraction. Their concentration is then measured either colorimetrically or spectrophotometrically. Spectrophotometric methods often rely on the reaction of alkaloids with specific reagents, such as bromocresol green (BCG), to form a colored product whose absorbance intensity is directly proportional to the alkaloid concentration.

**Procedure (Spectrophotometric Method using Bromocresol Green - BCG):**

1. **Plant Material Preparation:** The herbal raw material (e.g., *Tridax procumbens* leaves, or ingredients of Chitrakadivati) is ground into a fine powder.
2. **Extraction:** A quantity of 100 g of the ground plant material is extracted with methanol for 24 hours using a continuous extraction (Soxhlet) apparatus. The extract is then filtered, and the methanol is evaporated on a rotary evaporator under vacuum at a temperature of 45°C to yield a dry extract.
3. **Qualitative Test (Optional but Recommended):** To confirm the presence of alkaloids, a qualitative test, such as Dragendorff's method, is often performed. A portion of the extract is dissolved in dilute HCl, and two drops of Dragendorff's reagent are added. The formation of a crystalline precipitate indicates the presence of alkaloids.
4. **Reagent Preparation:**

- **Bromocresol Green (BCG) Solution:** 69.8 mg of bromocresol green is heated with 3 mL of 2N NaOH and 5 mL of distilled water until completely dissolved. The solution is then diluted to 1000 mL with distilled water.

- **Phosphate Buffer (pH 4.7):** The pH of a 2M sodium phosphate solution (71.6 gm $Na_2HPO_4$ in 1 L distilled water) is adjusted to 4.7 using 0.2 M citric acid (42.02 gm citric acid in 1 L distilled water).
- **Atropine Standard Solution:** A standard solution is prepared by dissolving 1 mg of pure Atropine (AR-grade) in 10 mL of distilled water.

5. **Quantitative Measurement:** The method relies on the reaction between the alkaloid and BCG, which forms a yellow-colored product. The concentration of this product is quantified either colorimetrically or using a UV-Spectrophotometer.
6. **Standard Curve:** A calibration curve is generated by measuring the absorbance of various known concentrations of a standard alkaloid (e.g., Atropine)
7. **Sample Measurement:** The absorbance of the prepared plant extract is measured under the same conditions.
8. **Calculation:** The total alkaloid content in the sample is determined by comparing its absorbance to the established standard curve.

**Precautions:**

- Methanol is a flammable and toxic solvent; therefore, all procedures involving methanol should be conducted in a fume hood.
- Sodium hydroxide (NaOH) is corrosive and handled carefully.
- All reagents should be handled with appropriate personal protective equipment (PPE).
- Proper disposal of organic waste is also essential.

**Result:** Alkaloid Content in Herbal Raw Materials was estimated.

## EXPERIMENT No: 16

**Object:** Estimation of flavonoid content in herbal raw materials.

**Requirements:**

**Reagents**: Herbal material, Ethanol (40%, 60%, 80% v/v), Aluminum chloride (AlCl3; 5.0% w/v in methanol), Rutin standard, Quercetin standard.

**Equipment:** Reflux apparatus, Volumetric flasks, Spectrophotometer, Pipettes, Cotton filter.

**Principles:** The quantification of flavonoids is commonly based on their ability to form colored complexes with aluminum chloride (AlCl3), which can then be measured using UV-Vis spectrophotometry. The intensity of the color formed is directly proportional to the concentration of flavonoids present.

**Procedure (UV-Vis Spectrophotometric Method using AlCl3):**

1. **Extract Preparation:** A quantity of 0.5 g of the herbal material (HM) is refluxed with 30 mL of 80% ethanol (v/v) at 85°C for 30 minutes. The extract is then filtered into a 100 mL volumetric flask. This extraction process is repeated twice more, each time with 15 mL of 80% ethanol for 15 minutes. The filtrates are collected, and the volume is made up to 100 mL with 80% ethanol. This serves as the stock solution.
2. **Standard and Sample Solutions:** Stock solutions of flavonoid standards (e.g., rutin, quercetin) are prepared in 50% ethanol (e.g., at concentrations of 0.10 mg/mL and 0.05 mg/mL, respectively). Aliquots of the HM stock solution (e.g., 3-6 mL) are transferred to 25 mL volumetric flasks.
3. **Complexation with AlCl3:** To the sample and standard aliquots in the volumetric flasks, 2 mL of AlCl3 solution (5.0%, w/v in methanol) is added. The volume is then made up with 50% ethanol.
4. **Reaction Time:** A reaction time of 25-30 minutes is allowed for the complexation to complete. The kinetics of the reaction can be further investigated by determining absorbances every 5 minutes for a total of 60 minutes.

5. **Absorbance Measurement:** The UV-Vis spectra are measured in the range of 300-500 nm using a spectrophotometer. The maximum absorption wavelength (λmax) is identified (e.g., 408 nm or 425 nm).
6. **Standard Curve & Calculation:** A standard curve is prepared by plotting the absorbance values of known standard concentrations against their respective concentrations. The total flavonoid content (TFC) of the sample is then expressed as g% of rutin or quercetin equivalents, based on this standard curve.

**Precautions:**

- All procedures should be conducted in a fume hood with appropriate personal protective equipment (PPE). Proper disposal of chemical waste is essential.

**Result:** Flavonoid content in herbal raw materials was estimated.

# EXPERIMENT No: 17

**Object:** Estimation of pesticidal residue in natural products with different analytical methods.

**Requirements:**

**Reagents:** Solvents (acetonitrile), Salts (magnesium sulfate, sodium acetate), Sorbents, Pesticide standards, Internal standards.

**Equipment:** Homogenizer, Centrifuge, GC-MS/MS system, LC-MS/MS system, Chromatographic columns, Various glassware for sample preparation.

**Principles:** Pesticides encompass a diverse array of organic compounds, each possessing unique physicochemical properties, including varying polarity, solubility, volatility, and stability. To efficiently analyze these complex mixtures, multiresidue methods, which allow for the simultaneous determination of multiple analytes, are preferred for their time and

cost-effectiveness. Gas Chromatography-Tandem Mass Spectrometry (GC-MS/MS) and Liquid Chromatography-Tandem Mass Spectrometry (LC-MS/MS) are the preferred analytical techniques due to their enhanced sensitivity and selectivity, particularly in the presence of co-eluting matrix interferences often encountered in natural product samples.

**Procedure** Sample Preparation :

**Homogenization:** The natural product is first homogenized (e.g., by cutting, grinding, or milling) to obtain a representative and homogeneous sample for analysis.

**Extraction:** Pesticide residues are isolated from the homogenized sample. This approach is a commonly used method, involving extraction with acetonitrile and salting out with magnesium sulfate and sodium acetate.

**Cleanup:** Co-extracted matrix components that could interfere with the analytical determination are removed. This often involves dispersive solid phase extraction (dSPE) using sorbents like primary secondary amine (PSA) to selectively remove sugars, fatty acids, and chlorophyll.

**1. Analysis by GC-MS/MS:**

**Instrumentation:** Agilent triple quadrupole GC/MS/MS systems are commonly recommended for this analysis. The system is typically equipped with a suitable chromatographic column (e.g., HP-5MS).

**Injection:** The cleaned extract is injected into the gas chromatograph.

**Separation:** Volatile pesticides are separated based on their boiling points and their interaction with the GC column.

**Detection:** The separated compounds are then detected by the mass spectrometry (MS/MS) system, which provides enhanced sensitivity and selectivity for their identification and quantification. Data is often acquired in selected-ion monitoring (SIM) mode for targeted analysis.

**2. Analysis by LC-MS/MS:**

- **Instrumentation:** LC-MS/MS systems (e.g., from Thermo Fisher Scientific) are utilized. Ultra-High Pressure Liquid Chromatography (UHPLC) coupled with High Resolution Accurate Mass (HRAM) technology is particularly effective for rapid and sensitive screening of both targeted and non-targeted pesticides.
- **Separation:** The liquid chromatograph (LC or UHPLC) separates pesticides based on their polarity using reversed-phase columns (e.g., C18, or aqueous C18 columns for more polar analytes).
- **Detection:** The MS/MS component provides highly selective and sensitive quantification and confirmation of hundreds of target pesticides in a single run.

**3. Data Processing:** The acquired data from either GC-MS/MS or LC-MS/MS is processed and analyzed to identify and quantify the pesticide residues present.

**4. Recovery Check:** The accuracy of the method is typically verified by spiking known concentrations of pesticides onto the surface of the sample or directly into the extract to determine recovery rates.

**Precautions:**

- Pesticides are inherently toxic compounds. Therefore, samples and standards must be handled with extreme care, using appropriate personal protective equipment (PPE) such as gloves, lab coats, and eye protection, and working exclusively within a fume hood.

- Proper disposal of all hazardous chemical waste is critically important to prevent environmental contamination and exposure.

**Result:** Pesticidal residue in natural products with different analytical methods was estimated.

## EXPERIMENT No: 12

**Object:** In vitro antidiabetic screening of Plant Extracts (Alpha-Amylase and Alpha-Glucosidase Inhibition Assays).

**Requirements:**

**Reagents:** Plant extracts, Dimethyl sulfoxide (DMSO), Potato starch, 3,5-dinitrosalicylic acid (DNSA), Sodium potassium tartrate, Sodium hydroxide, Sodium phosphate buffer (pH 6.9), Hydrochloric acid, Distilled water, Alpha-amylase, Sodium chloride, p-nitrophenyl glucopyranoside (pNPG), Alpha-glucosidase, Commercial kit components (Acarbose, alpha-Glucosidase Positive Control, Assay Buffer, Substrate Mix).

**Equipment:** Conviron system, Electric grinder, Shaker, Sonication bath, Centrifuge, Filter paper, Vials, Magnetic stirrer, Hot plate, Dark glass bottle, Hot water bath, spectrophotometer, Microplate reader.

**Principles:**

Alpha-amylase, which is in saliva and pancreatic juice, breaks down big starch molecules into smaller ones that can be absorbed. Alpha-glucosidase, which is found in the brush border of the small intestine, breaks down disaccharides and oligosaccharides into glucose even more. Inhibitors of these enzymes slow down the absorption of glucose, which is a good way to keep blood glucose levels in check for people with diabetes. Researchers are actively looking for natural sources of these inhibitors to find alternatives that may have fewer side effects than synthetic drugs.

**Procedure (Alpha-Amylase Inhibitory Assay):**

1. **Sample Preparation:** Plant extracts (e.g., leaf, stem, root extracts) are dried. Aqueous extracts are often lyophilized, while solvent-extracted residues are dissolved in a suitable solvent like 10% dimethyl sulfoxide (DMSO). All extracts are standardized to a specific concentration (e.g., 100 mg/ml), and serial dilutions are prepared in triplicate across a relevant concentration range (e.g., 20 to 100 mg/ml).
2. **Enzyme Solution Preparation:** An alpha-amylase solution (e.g., 2 units/ml) is prepared by dissolving the enzyme (e.g., from *Aspergillus oryzae*) in a 0.02 M sodium phosphate buffer (pH 6.9) containing 6.7 mM sodium chloride.

3. **Pre-incubation:** A specified volume of plant extract (e.g., 500 μl) is incubated with an equal volume of alpha-amylase solution for 10 minutes at room temperature (e.g., 32°C or 25°C).
4. **Substrate Addition:** After pre-incubation, a 1% starch solution (prepared by mixing starch with distilled water, heating, and stirring) is added to the mixture at timed intervals (e.g., 500 μl).
5. **Second Incubation:** The combined solution is further incubated for another 10 minutes at the same temperature.
6. **Reaction Termination:** The enzymatic reaction is terminated by adding a specific volume (e.g., 1 ml or 500 μl) of 3,5-dinitrosalicylic acid (DNSA) reagent. The mixture is then incubated in a hot water bath (e.g., 85°C or boiling water) for 5 minutes. The termination is indicated by a visible color change to orange-red
7. **Cooling and Volume Adjustment:** The mixture is removed from the hot water bath, allowed to cool to room temperature, and the volume is adjusted (e.g., to 5 ml) with distilled water.
8. **Blank and Control Experiments:** Blank experiments are conducted by substituting the enzyme with buffer, while the plant extract itself can serve as a positive control. A control without extract (only solvent with enzyme) is also necessary.
9. **Absorbance Measurement:** The absorbance of the resulting solution is measured at 540 nm using a spectrometer.
10. **Inhibition Calculation:** The percentage of inhibition is calculated using a formula, and the concentration of extracts resulting in 50% inhibition of enzyme activity (IC50) is determined graphically.

**Procedure (Alpha-Glucosidase Inhibitory Assay):**

1. **Substrate Solution Preparation:** The substrate p-nitrophenyl glucopyranoside (pNPG) is prepared in a 20 mM phosphate buffer (pH 6.9).
2. **Pre-incubation:** A specified volume of alpha-glucosidase (e.g., 1.0 U/mL) is pre-incubated with various concentrations of the plant extracts (e.g., acetone, ethanol, water extracts) for 10 minutes.

3. **Substrate Addition:** A volume of 3.0 mM pNPG (dissolved in 20 mM phosphate buffer, pH 6.9) is added to initiate the reaction.
4. **Incubation:** The reaction mixture is incubated at 37°C for 20 minutes
5. **Reaction Termination:** The reaction is stopped by adding a specific volume (e.g., 2 mL) of 0.1 M Na2CO3.
6. **Absorbance Measurement:** The alpha-glucosidase activity is determined by measuring the yellow-colored paranitrophenol released from pNPG at 405 nm using a spectrophotometer.
7. **Inhibition Calculation:** Results are expressed as a percentage of the blank control, and the IC50 value is determined graphically.

**Precautions:**

- Standard laboratory safety practices must be followed, including the use of appropriate personal protective equipment (PPE), proper handling of chemical reagents, and sterile techniques to prevent contamination.

**Result:** In vitro antidiabetic screening of Plant Extracts (Alpha-Amylase and Alpha-Glucosidase Inhibition Assays) was performed.

## EXPERIMENT No: 19

**Object:** Isolation of Nucleic Acid from Cauliflower Heads (Genomic DNA).

**Requirements:**

**Reagents:**

- Cauliflower tissue
- CTAB Buffer
- RNase A solution
- Phenol/chloroform/isoamyl alcohol (25:24:1)
- Cold isopropanol
- Ice-cold 70% ethanol
- TE buffer (10 mM Tris, pH 8, 1 mM EDTA)
- For Synergy™ protocol: Synergy™ 2.0 Plant DNA Extraction kit

**Equipment:**

- Polypropylene tubes
- Water bath (60°C and 37°C)
- Centrifuge (14,000 x g)
- SpeedVac (optional)
- Microcentrifuge tubes
- Bead beater, silica spin columns

**Principles:** Cauliflower cells, like all plant cells, contain nucleic acids (mainly DNA) inside the nucleus. To isolate DNA, the cells must be lysed (broken open) to release their internal contents. The isolation process involves several key steps: 1) disruption of cells to release DNA from the nucleus, 2) inhibition of DNA-degrading enzymes (DNases) to protect the integrity of the DNA, 3) dissociation of DNA-protein complexes to separate DNA from associated proteins, 4) removal of contaminants such as proteins, polysaccharides, and other cellular debris, and 5) precipitation of purified DNA from the solution.

**Procedure (CTAB Protocol):** The CTAB (Cetyltrimethylammonium Bromide) protocol is a common method for isolating genomic DNA from plant tissues.

1. **Tissue Grinding:** The cauliflower tissue is ground into a fine powder. This increases

the surface area for efficient cell lysis.

2. **Cell Lysis and Protein Dissociation:** For every 100 mg of homogenized tissue, 500 µl of CTAB Buffer is added to a polypropylene tube. The mixture is thoroughly vortexed and then incubated in a 60°C water bath for 30 minutes. CTAB is a detergent that helps disrupt cell membranes and dissociate DNA-protein complexes.
3. **Centrifugation:** The homogenate is centrifuged at 14,000 x g for 5 minutes to pellet cellular debris and insoluble material.
4. **RNase Treatment:** The supernatant, containing DNA and RNA, is transferred to a new tube. 5 µl of RNase A solution is added, and the mixture is incubated at 37°C for 20 minutes to degrade RNA.
5. **Phenol/Chloroform Extraction:** An equal volume of phenol/chloroform/isoamyl alcohol (25:24:1) is added. The mixture is vortexed for 5 seconds and then centrifuged at 14,000 x g for 1 minute to separate the aqueous (upper) and organic (lower) phases. The aqueous phase, containing the DNA, is transferred to a new tube. This extraction is repeated until the aqueous phase appears clear, indicating effective protein removal
6. **DNA Precipitation:** 0.7 volume of cold isopropanol is added to the aqueous phase, and the mixture is incubated at -20°C for 15 minutes to precipitate the DNA.
7. **DNA Pellet Collection:** The sample is centrifuged at 14,000 x g for 10 minutes to pellet the precipitated DNA.
8. **Ethanol Wash:** The supernatant is carefully decanted without disturbing the DNA pellet. The pellet is then washed with 500 µl of ice-cold 70% ethanol to remove residual salts and contaminants.
9. **Drying:** The ethanol is decanted, and residual ethanol is removed by drying the pellet in a SpeedVac or by air-drying. The pellet should be dried just enough to remove alcohol but not completely, to prevent irreversible denaturation.

10. **DNA Dissolution:** The DNA pellet is dissolved in 20 µl of TE buffer (10 mM Tris, pH 8, 1 mM EDTA). Warming may be necessary to facilitate dissolution.
11. **Optional Protocol (Synergy™ Protocol - Phenol/Chloroform-free):** This method eliminates the use of hazardous chemicals like phenol and chloroform but requires a bead beater for homogenization. It typically involves homogenization with a

specialized buffer, RNase treatment, and purification using silica spin columns.

**Precautions:**

- Phenol and chloroform are highly hazardous chemicals, therefore, all steps involving these reagents must be performed in a fume hood with appropriate personal protective equipment (PPE), including chemical-resistant gloves and eye protection.
- Ethanol and isopropanol are flammable and should be handled away from ignition sources.
- Proper disposal of hazardous chemical waste is mandatory.

**Result:** Nucleic Acid from Cauliflower Heads was isolated.

# EXPERIMENT No: 20

**Object:** Isolation of RNA from Yeast.

**Requirements:**

**Reagents:**

- Yeast cells
- Desired growth medium
- TES solution
- Acid phenol (pH 5)
- SDS
- Chloroform
- 3 M sodium acetate (pH 5.3)
- 100% and 70% ice-cold ethanol
- Nuclease-free water
- For SV system: SV RNA Lysis Buffer, SV RNA Dilution Buffer, Lyticase (or Zymolase), 1M sorbitol, 0.1M EDTA (pH 8.0), 0.1% beta-mercaptoethanol

**Equipment:**

- Centrifuge tubes
- Tabletop centrifuge or microcentrifuge
- Water bath
- Vortexer
- Liquid nitrogen
- Spectrophotometer

**Principles:** RNA isolation involves efficient cell lysis to release nucleic acids, followed by the removal of contaminating macromolecules like DNA and proteins, and finally, the precipitation and purification of the RNA. The integrity of RNA is highly susceptible to degradation by ubiquitous RNases, making rapid and careful handling essential.

**Procedure (Hot Acidic Phenol Extraction):** This method is highly efficient for isolating RNA directly from intact yeast cells.

**Yeast Culture Preparation:** Grow an overnight culture of yeast in an appropriate medium and at the correct temperature. Dilute the overnight culture (e.g., 1:50) and grow to mid-exponential phase (OD600 = 0.5-1.0). RNA yields are less consistent from stationary phase cultures.

1. **Cell Pellet Collection:** Transfer the culture to a 50-mL centrifuge tube and centrifuge cells at 1500 x g (7000 rpm in a tabletop centrifuge or SS-34 rotor) for 3 minutes at 4°C.
2. **Pellet Resuspension:** Discard the supernatant and resuspend the pellet in 1 mL of ice-cold water. Transfer to a clean 1.5-mL microcentrifuge tube, microcentrifuge for 10 seconds at 4°C, and remove the supernatant. The pellet can be frozen in liquid nitrogen and stored at -70°C for months if desired.
3. **Lysis and Phenol Extraction (First Round):** Resuspend the cell pellet in 400 µl of TES solution. Add 400 µl of acid phenol (preheated to 65°C) and vortex vigorously for 10 seconds. Incubate at 65°C for 60 minutes, with brief vortexing for 10 seconds every 15 minutes. Incubation for at least 30 minutes is crucial for quantitative recovery.
4. **Phase Separation (First Round):** Place the tube on ice for 5 minutes. Microcentrifuge for 5 minutes at top speed at 4°C.
5. **Phenol Extraction (Second Round):** Transfer the aqueous (top) phase to a clean 1.5-mL microcentrifuge tube. Add 400 µl of acid phenol and vortex vigorously. Repeat the centrifugation step from step 5.
6. **Chloroform Extraction:** Transfer the aqueous phase to a new 1.5-mL microcentrifuge tube. Add 400 µl of chloroform, vortex vigorously, and microcentrifuge for 5 minutes at top speed at 4°C. This step helps remove residual phenol.
7. **RNA Precipitation:** Transfer the aqueous phase to a new tube. Add 40 µl of 3 M sodium acetate (pH 5.3) and 1 mL of ice-cold 100% ethanol. RNA is usually precipitated overnight at -20°C or -70°C.

8. **RNA Pellet Wash:** Microcentrifuge for 5 minutes at top speed at 4°C to pellet the RNA. Wash the RNA pellet by briefly vortexing in ice-cold 70% ethanol. Microcentrifuge again to re-pellet the RNA. The long centrifugation in this step helps dry the spin column membrane, preventing ethanol carryover that could interfere with downstream reactions.
9. **Drying and Resuspension:** Dry the RNA pellet by keeping the tube open for approximately 10 minutes. Resuspend the pellet in 50 µl of nuclease-free water. If necessary, heat at 65°C for 10-20 minutes or dilute further to ensure complete dissolution.
10. **Concentration Determination:** Determine the RNA concentration

spectrophotometrically by measuring absorbance at A260 and A280.

**Precautions:**

- All procedures involving these chemicals must be performed in a fume hood with appropriate personal protective equipment (PPE), including chemical-resistant gloves and eye protection.
- Liquid nitrogen requires specific handling precautions due to extreme cold.
- Strict adherence to aseptic techniques is crucial throughout the process to prevent RNA degradation by ubiquitous RNases.

**Result:** RNA from Yeast was isolated.

# EXPERIMENT No: 21

**Object:** Quantitative estimation of DNA by the spectrophotometric method.

**Requirements:**

**Equipment:** Spectrophotometer, Cuvettes and Pipettes

**Principle:** DNA strongly absorbs ultraviolet (UV) radiation at a wavelength of 260 nm. This absorbance is primarily due to the conjugated bonding systems of the purine and pyrimidine bases (adenine, guanine, cytosine, thymine) that constitute DNA. The Beer-Lambert law applies

to this absorption, allowing for the calculation of DNA concentration based on its absorbance.

**Procedure:**

1. **Sample Preparation:** The DNA sample is prepared, typically dissolved in distilled water or saline.
2. **Absorbance Measurement:** A 3 mL aliquot of the given DNA sample is pipetted into a cuvette. The absorbance is then measured at 260 nm (A260) against a blank of distilled water or saline. For accurate readings, the absorbance at 260 nm should ideally fall between 0.15 and 1.0.
3. **Concentration Calculation:** The concentration of DNA in the sample is calculated using a conversion factor. Theoretically, one optical density (OD) unit at 260 nm corresponds to 50 μg/mL for double-stranded DNA (dsDNA) and 33 μg/mL for single-stranded DNA (ssDNA).

   - The formula for dsDNA is: DNA concentration (μg/mL) = Absorbance at 260 × 50.

4. **Purity Assessment (Optional but Recommended):** The purity of the DNA sample is often assessed by calculating the A260/A280 ratio. For pure DNA, this ratio should be between 1.8 and 2.0 in 10 mM Tris·Cl, pH 8.5. A ratio significantly lower than 1.8 may indicate protein contamination, while a higher ratio could suggest RNA contamination.

**Precautions:**

- General laboratory safety practices, including proper handling of samples and glassware, should be followed. UV light from the spectrophotometer should not be directly viewed.

**Result:** Quantitative estimation of DNA by the spectrophotometric method was done.

# EXPERIMENT No: 22

**Object:** Immobilization of Whole Cell (Alginate Bead Protocol).

**Requirements:**

**Reagents:**

- Sodium alginate
- Calcium chloride
- Xanthan gum
- Surfactant
- Process buffer
- Culture medium
- Calcium carbonate powder
- Acetic acid
- Mineral oil

**Equipment:**

- Nozzles
- Stirred vessel
- Magnetic stir plate
- Rotary mixer
- Autoclave
- Conical tubes
- Fume hood
- Pipettes

**Principles:** Cell immobilization in alginate beads is primarily achieved through cell entrapment within a gel matrix. This process typically relies on ionotropic gelation, where a solution containing cells and sodium alginate forms beads upon contact with a solution containing divalent cations, most commonly calcium chloride (CaCl2). These cations diffuse into the alginate droplets, causing the alginate polymer to cross-link and form a stable gel. An alternative method is internal gelation, which involves creating a water-in-oil emulsion of alginate droplets containing a fine-grain calcium salt, followed by the addition of acid to trigger gelation from within the droplets.

**Procedure (External Gelation - Common for Microbial Cells):**

1. **Cell-Alginate Mixture:** Whole microbial cells are thoroughly mixed with a sodium alginate solution. A small amount of xanthan gum may be added to improve the properties of the mixture.
2. **Bead Formation:** The resultant mixture is added drop-wise, while stirring, into a CaCl2 solution. As the droplets fall into the calcium chloride, they instantly gel

to form spherical alginate beads containing the entrapped cells. A small amount of surfactant (preferably polyoxyethylenesorbitan monolaurate) may be included in the Na-alginate solution to obtain perfectly spherical capsules.

3. **Washing and Hardening:** The newly formed alginate beads are washed with distilled water to remove excess CaCl2 and then further hardened by incubation in a fresh CaCl2 solution.

4. **Incubation:** The hardened beads are then transferred to an appropriate growth medium for the immobilized cells.

**Procedure (Internal Gelation for Mammalian Cells - More Complex):** This method is particularly useful for achieving high-concentration alginate beads and involves more intricate preparation steps.

1. **Prepare Alginate Solution, CaCO3 Suspension, and Acidified Oil:**

- **Alginate Solution:** Prepare a stock solution of sodium alginate (e.g., 5% alginate) in a process buffer (e.g., 10 mM HEPES, 170 mM NaCl, pH 7.4). Weigh the alginate powder and progressively add it to the stirring buffer, allowing it to dissolve overnight. Sterilize by autoclaving.
- **CaCO3 Suspension:** Prepare a calcium carbonate (CaCO3) suspension in process buffer (e.g., 24 mM CaCO3). Autoclave for sterilization.
- **Acidified Oil:** Immediately before emulsification, dissolve acetic acid (e.g., 44 μL) in mineral oil (e.g., 11 mL) in a conical tube. Ensure complete dissolution by repeated.

2. **Cell Encapsulation (Emulsification and Gelation):**

- The encapsulant (e.g., mammalian cells) is dispersed in the alginate solution, which also contains a fine-grain calcium salt with low solubility at the initial process pH.
- This alginate mixture is then added to an agitated organic phase (mineral oil with surfactant) to create a water-in-oil emulsion.
- Acetic acid, added to the organic phase, is transported to the alginate droplets. It partitions into the aqueous phase, dissociates, and diffuses to the CaCO3, causing internal gelation of the alginate droplets.

3. **Post-Encapsulation:** The capsules may be washed with distilled water, hardened in a CaCl2 solution, and incubated in a growth medium.

**Precautions:**

- Acetic acid is a toxic and volatile acid; it must be handled under a fume hood, and its solutions should be kept in closed containers until the emulsification step.
- Autoclaving procedures require careful adherence to safety protocols. General sterile techniques are crucial for all cell culture work to prevent contamination.

**Result:** Immobilization of Whole Cell (Alginate Bead Protocol) was performed.

# EXPERIMENT No: 23

**Object:** Establishment of Callus Culture.

**Requirements:**

**Reagents:**

- Plant explants
- Surface sterilants
- Culture medium components
- Plant growth regulators
- Sterile distilled water

**Equipment:**

- Petri dishes or other closed culture vessels
- Laminar flow hood
- Scalpel
- Beakers
- Detergent
- Shaker
- Drying oven
- Autoclave

**Principles:** Callus formation is initiated by stimulating the dedifferentiation and subsequent proliferation of plant cells. This process is primarily triggered by a specific balance of plant growth regulators, particularly auxins and cytokinins, supplied in a nutrient-rich culture medium. The precise ratio of these hormones is critical for inducing the desired unorganized growth.

**Procedure:**

1. **Explant Selection & Surface Sterilization:** Appropriate plant tissues (explants), such as leaf fragments, roots, or stems, are selected. These explants must undergo rigorous surface sterilization to eliminate dirt, bacteria, fungi, and other contaminants that could compromise the culture.

- **Initial Wash:** Explants can be washed in soapy water, followed by running tap water for 1-2 hours, and then distilled water to remove external debris.
- **Disinfection:** A common method involves surface disinfection with 70% ethanol for a brief period (a few seconds to minutes), followed by treatment with a disinfectant solution like sodium hypochlorite (bleach, diluted to 0.5-1.0% for 10-20 minutes) or calcium hypochlorite. Mercuric chloride and hydrogen peroxide are also effective but are highly toxic and used rarely.
- **Rinsing:** After disinfectant treatment, explants are rinsed multiple times with sterile distilled water to remove all traces of the sterilant, as residues can be phytotoxic.
- **Trimming:** The explants are then trimmed to the desired size using a sharp scalpel under sterile conditions, typically within a laminar flow hood.

2. **Media Preparation:** Callus induction medium is prepared. This medium typically consists of agar (as a solidifying agent), a mixture of macronutrients and micronutrients (e.g., modified Murashige and Skoog medium, White's medium, or woody plant medium), and vitamins (e.g., Gamborg B5 vitamins) to enhance growth. Crucially, plant growth regulators, such as auxins (e.g., 2,4-D, NAA, IAA) and cytokinins (e.g., BA), are added. The specific ratio of auxin to cytokinin is paramount; for instance, a higher auxin-to-cytokinin ratio generally promotes rooting, while equal amounts stimulate callus growth, and a higher cytokinin ratio promotes shoot

development

3. **Inoculation:** The surface-sterilized explants are aseptically plated onto the prepared gel medium within a closed culture vessel, such as a Petri dish.
4. **Incubation:** The cultures are typically incubated in the dark at a controlled temperature, commonly 25°C.

5. **Subculture:** Once callus has formed, it is separated from the original explant and repeatedly subcultured onto fresh medium (e.g., every 30 days) to maintain vigorous growth and obtain friable callus suitable for further applications.

**Precautions:**

- Mercuric chloride and hydrogen peroxide are highly dangerous chemicals and should be handled with extreme caution.
- Strict aseptic techniques are paramount throughout the entire process to prevent microbial contamination, which can rapidly destroy cultures.

**Result:** Callus Culture was established.

# EXPERIMENT No: 24

**Object:** Establishment of Suspension Culture.

**Requirements:**

**Reagents:**

- Friable callus
- Liquid MS medium
- NAA (Naphthaleneacetic acid)
- BA (Benzyladenine)
- Sucrose
- Sterile water
- Optional: B5 vitamin stock, other growth regulator stocks

**Equipments:**

- Erlenmeyer flasks
- Shaker
- Inoculated spatula or tweezers
- Pipettes
- Sieves
- Sterile culture bottles

**Principle:**

Suspension cultures are usually started with friable callus, which is then moved to a liquid medium. Constant shaking or oscillation gives a gentle rheological force that breaks up cell clusters into smaller aggregates and single cells, which helps them spread out evenly in the medium. This agitation also makes it easier for substances to move between the medium and the cells, and it makes it easier for gases to move between the air and the liquid, which makes sure that there is enough oxygen for breathing and that carbon dioxide is removed quickly, all of which help cells grow quickly.

**Procedure:**

1. **Callus Induction & Domestication:** The prerequisite for establishing a suspension culture is a well-established, friable callus culture (as described in Section 9.2). The callus should be in a vigorous growth phase, characterized by fast-growing, fresh, young, small, loose, friable, moist-looking, uniform, white, or pale yellow appearance.
2. **Inoculation of Callus:** A quantity of approximately 3 g of white and friable callus (or about 2 g of loose and fragile callus in its vigorous growth phase) is aseptically transferred into a 250 mL Erlenmeyer flask containing 100 mL of fresh liquid

Murashige and Skoog (MS) medium. The liquid medium components are generally the same as those used for callus induction, but without agar. This medium is typically supplemented with plant growth regulators such as NAA (0.5 mg/l), BA (2.0 mg/l), and sucrose (30 g/l), with the pH adjusted to 5.8. An inoculated spatula or tweezers are used to gently break up the callus mass within the liquid medium.

3. **Shaking Culture:** The Erlenmeyer flask is sealed and placed on a shaker, typically set at 120 revolutions per minute (r/min), and incubated at 25°C in the dark. The continuous oscillation is vital for disaggregating cell clusters and maintaining a homogeneous suspension.
4. **Subculture:** Suspension cultures are subcultured regularly, typically every 7 or 14 days. During subculture, the culture bottle is allowed to stand still for a period, allowing larger cell clusters to settle at the bottom. The cell suspension from the middle of the flask is then pipetted into a new culture flask, and 2-4 times the volume of fresh medium is added. For a more homogeneous starting material, cells can be sieved sequentially through 850 μm and 500 μm sieves.
5. **Maintenance:** The cell suspensions are sieved and subcultured every 7 days until a homogeneous proliferating cell population is firmly established

**Precautions:**

- Strict aseptic conditions are critically important throughout the entire process to prevent microbial contamination. This includes flaming the neck of flasks before opening them and constantly swirling the flask and moving the pipette to avoid clogging.
- Regular checks for bacterial and/or fungal contamination by plating aliquots on growth media are recommended.

**Result:** Suspension Culture was established.

# EXPERIMENT No: 25

**Object:** Preparation and Standardization of Various Simple Dosage Forms from Ayurvedic, Siddha, Homoeopathy, and Unani Formulary.

**Requirements:**

Preparation of these traditional dosage forms often involves traditional vessels (e.g., wooden barrels, earthen pots, closed crucibles) alongside modern laboratory equipment for powdering, mixing, heating, and filtration. For standardization, analytical instruments such as pH meters, balances, dissolution testers, and hardness testers are employed.

**Theory:**

Making and standardizing traditional dosage forms from Ayurvedic, Siddha, Homoeopathy, and Unani systems of medicine is very important for making sure that they are safe, effective, and of high quality in modern pharmaceutical practice. This process combines old-fashioned wisdom with modern analytical rigor.

**Ayurvedic Dosage Forms:** Ayurvedic formulations are broadly categorized into solid, semi-solid, liquid, and powder forms, utilizing ingredients from plant, animal, and mineral origins.

1. **Aristas and Asavas (Fermented Liquid Preparations):**
    - **Preparation:** These are self-generated alcoholic preparations. Aristas are made from the decoction (Kashaya) of crude drugs, while Asavas involve directly adding powdered drugs to a solution of sugar or jaggery. The mixture is boiled, cooled, and transferred to wooden barrels or earthen pots for fermentation (Sandhana). The containers are sealed and kept in an underground cellar or paddy heap to maintain a constant temperature. After the specified fermentation period, the fluid is filtered and stored.
    - **Standardization:** Parameters include organoleptic characteristics (color, odor, taste), physical properties (pH, moisture content, melting/boiling point, refractive index, specific gravity, alcohol content, extractive value), and chemical composition

(alkaloids, glycosides, flavonoids, phenols, tannins).

2. **Vati and Ghutika (Tablets and Pills - Solid Dosage Forms):**

   **Preparation:** Drugs are dried and finely powdered. Mineral drugs are converted into calcined products (bhasmas) or other specified forms. All ingredients are mixed according to the formula, and a soft paste is prepared using specified liquids. This paste is then ground and formed into tablets (vati) or pills (ghutika). Heat-processed vati (Sagnisadhya Vati) involves melting jaggery, sugar, or guggulu with powdered herbs before shaping.

   **Standardization:** Key parameters include uniformity of weight, hardness, disintegration time, water-soluble extract, alcohol-soluble extract, ash value, and loss on drying. Physical characteristics such as bulk density, tapped density, angle of repose, Hausner ratio, and Carr's index are also evaluated for powder flowability. pH and solubility tests are also performed.

3. **Churna (Powder Dosage Forms):**

   **Preparation:** Single or combined drugs are separately dried, finely powdered, and sieved to ensure uniform particle size. These are then mixed to obtain a homogeneous powder.

   **Standardization:** Parameters include pH, moisture content, ash value, and extractive value.

4. **Leham (Semi-solid Dosage Forms):**

   **Preparation:** Also known as Avaleha, these are semisolid preparations made by boiling powdered drugs or extracts with a solution of sugar or jaggery. Powdered drugs/extracts and other ingredients are added with continuous stirring to form a homogeneous semisolid mass. Ghee or oil may be added while the preparation is hot.

   **Standardization:** Organoleptic properties (color, odor, taste) and physical parameters (pH, moisture content, loss on drying, refractive index, specific gravity, alcohol content, extractive value) are assessed.

5. **Bhasmas (Calcined Minerals/Metals - Powdered Forms):**

- **Preparation (Two Stages):**

1. **Sodhana (Purification):** Metals and minerals undergo purification by heating and immersing them in specific liquids to remove toxicity.

2. **Marana (Second Stage):** The purified drugs are ground and mixed with specified plants or extracts. Small cakes are formed, sun-dried, placed in sealed earthen vessels, and heated in a pit covered with cow dung. After heating for a specified period, the contents are removed, ground into a fine powder, and stored.

- **Standardization:** Bhasmas are typically grey, whitish, yellowish, or black powders. They should retain their color upon storage and remain highly stable, preserving their potency over long periods.

**A. Siddha System:**

**Dosage Forms:** Include Kudineer (herbal decoction), Chooranam (herbal powder), Mathirai/Vatakam (tablets), Legiyam (herbal electuary), Thylam (medicated oil), and mineral/metal preparations like Parpam, Chendooram, and Mezhugu.

- **Preparation (Gunapadam):** This branch focuses on the qualities, properties, preparation, purification, dosage, and therapeutic application of drugs.

**Purification (Suddhi):** Raw drugs, particularly metals and minerals, undergo purification using herbal juices, lime water, or cow's urine to remove toxicity, impurities, and enhance therapeutic potency. Common methods include trituration (for mercury), melting and pouring into liquid (for sulfur), and boiling with herbal juices (for arsenicals, iron, copper).

**Incineration (Maruthuvam):** Used for preparing mineral/metal-based formulations like Parpam and Chendooram, involving controlled heating in earthen pots.

**Grinding (Kalvam):** Utilizes stone grinders with herbal liquids to increase drug potency and bioavailability.

- **Standardization:** Siddha formulations adhere to pharmacopoeial standards (e.g., Pharmacopoeial Standards for Siddha Formulations (PCIM&H), Siddha Pharmacopoeia of India). Standardization includes physicochemical parameters (pH, viscosity, specific gravity, loss on drying, acid value, saponification value, peroxide value, iodine value, refractive index, rancidity), phytochemical screening (tannins, phenols, terpenoids, alkaloids, flavonoids, carbohydrates), and microbial load testing. HPTLC fingerprinting is also utilized.

**B. Unani System:**

- **Dosage Forms:** Encompass Jawarish/Majoon (semi-solid herbal pastes), Khamira (syrupy semi-solids), Sufuf (powders), Qurs/Hab (tablets or pills), Sharbat (syrups),

Tiryaq/Laooq (electuaries/confections), Arq (distillates), and Zamad/Marham (external pastes and ointments).

- **Preparation and Standardization:** While the existence of these dosage forms implies established preparation methods, detailed protocols for Unani formulations are not provided in the snippets. However, physicochemical analysis and phytochemical screening are general quality control measures applicable to all traditional systems of medicine.

C. **Homoeopathy System:**

- **Dosage Forms:** Include Dilutions (potencies, alcohol-based solutions), Medicated Globules (sucrose or lactose pellets), Tablets, Mother Tinctures (original extracts), Ointments/Creams, and External Drops.
- **Preparation:** The fundamental principle is "Potentization," which involves serial dilution and succussion (vigorous shaking) to enhance the energetic properties of the remedy.

**Precautions:**

Proper handling of raw materials, particularly ensuring that purification steps (e.g., Sodhana in Ayurveda, Suddhi in Siddha) are meticulously followed for toxic ingredients (e.g., metals, minerals), is critical to ensure the safety of the final product.

**Result:** Various Simple Dosage Forms from Ayurvedic, Siddha, Homoeopathy, and Unani Formulary was prepared and standardized.

# EXPERIMENT No: 26

**Object:** Preparation of certain Aromatherapy Formulations.

**Requirements:**

**Reagents:**

- Selected essential oils
- Carrier oils for topical application

**Equipment:**

- Perfume strips (aroma wands)
- Empty dark glass bottles with caps
- Pipettes or droppers

**Theory:** Aromatherapy formulations involve the skillful blending of essential oils to create specific therapeutic or sensory experiences. This process combines an understanding of aromatic properties with precise formulation principles.

**Principle:** Essential oil blending is based on the concept of aromatic notes and aroma strength. Essential oils are categorized into three main notes based on their volatility and persistence:

a. **Top Notes:** These are the first noticeable impressions in a blend, characterized by a swift, sharp aroma that evaporates quickly (e.g., Bergamot, Lemon, Sweet Orange, Eucalyptus, Sage).

b. **Middle Notes:** These oils bind the entire blend together, providing a consistent and often strong central aroma that lasts longer than top notes (e.g., Lavender, Geranium, Cinnamon, Tea Tree, Rosemary).

c. **Base Notes:** These are the slowest to evaporate, providing depth and grounding to the blend, and are the last scents to dissipate (e.g., Cedarwood, Frankincense, Patchouli, Vetiver, Peppermint). Creating a blend with a tiered selection of notes (top, middle, base) ensures a longer-lasting and evolving aroma. For topical application, essential oils are always diluted in a carrier oil.

**Procedure:**

1. **Essential Oil Selection:** Begin by choosing essential oils that are believed to create a pleasant and desired aromatherapy blend. This selection often involves reflecting on naturally enjoyable fragrances and performing organoleptic tests on the chosen oils.
2. **Aromatic Notes Identification:** Identify the selected oils as top, middle, or base notes. Ideally, a blend will include at least two top notes, two middle notes, and one base note to create a balanced aroma.
3. **Aroma Strength Assessment:** Consider the individual aroma strength of each chosen oil, which is distinct from its evaporation rate. A very powerful aroma will require a smaller quantity in the blend to prevent it from dominating. For example, Roman chamomile has a much stronger aroma than lavender, so more lavender is needed to balance the blend (e.g., 4-8 drops of lavender to 1 drop of chamomile).
4. **Ratio Determination:** A good rule of thumb is to base the aromatherapy formula on a total of 100 drops to easily determine the percentage of each essential oil in the blend. Common blending ratios suggest 30% top notes, 50% middle notes, and 20% base notes for the final blend. For topical application, a typical dilution is 15 drops of essential oil per 30 mL of carrier oil.
5. **Blending:** Combine the selected essential oils in the determined ratios. This can be done by creating an "aroma wand" (a few drops of each oil on separate perfume strips) and wafting them to adjust ratios based on perceived aroma strength.

- **Storage:** To ensure the longevity and potency of the blended essential oil, it should be stored in dark glass bottles, tightly sealed to prevent oxidation, and kept away from direct sunlight and heat in a cool, dark place. Maintaining notes of preferred formulas is recommended for future reference. Pen and paper (for recording formulations).

**Result:** Aromatherapy Formulations was prepared.

# EXPERIMENT No: 27

**Object:** Formulation of Herbal Cosmetics (Lip Balm, Lipstick, Facial Cream, Herbal Hair and Nail Care Products).

**Requirements:**

Water bath, muslin cloth, china dish, storage containers, filter paper, pectin, citric acid, honey, castor oil, coconut oil, orange oil, distilled water, methanol, glycerine, potassium hydroxide, triethanolamine.

**Theory:** The formulation of herbal cosmetics, such as lip balms, lipsticks, facial creams, and various hair and nail care products, is driven by a growing consumer demand for natural, safe, and effective beauty solutions. These products aim to reduce toxicity and improve safety compared to synthetic counterparts, leveraging the inherent benefits of plant-based ingredients.

**A. Herbal Lip Balm Formulation:**

- **Ingredients:** The formulation typically includes a blend of natural waxes (e.g., Carnauba wax, Beeswax), butters (e.g., Shea butter, general butter), and oils (e.g., Coconut oil, Castor oil) for moisturizing and emollient properties. Active botanical extracts, such as Red Dragon Fruit (Hylocereus polyrhizus) for its antioxidant and natural colorant properties, and honey for its beneficial effects, are incorporated. Pectin and citric acid may be used in extract preparation, and orange oil can be added for flavor and skin benefits.
- **Procedure (Red Dragon Fruit Extract):** The flesh of red dragon fruit is sliced and boiled with water for 20-30 minutes. The extract is collected using a muslin cloth, re-boiled with stirring, and then pectin and citric acid are added. Any scum is removed, and the extract is transferred to a bottle.
- **Procedure (Lip Balm):** Waxes and butters are melted together in a china dish. The prepared red dragon fruit extract is added to the melted mixture. The dish is removed

from heat, and honey, castor oil, coconut oil, and orange oil are incorporated. The mixture is then poured into lip balm containers, sealed, and stored.

- **Evaluation:** The formulated lip balm undergoes evaluation for organoleptic properties (color, odor, appearance), melting point, pH, spreadability, and solubility. Microbial testing is performed to ensure safety (limit of not more than 100 colonies). An antioxidant test (observing time to darken) and stability studies (at room, refrigeration, and oven temperatures for 30 days) are also conducted.

**B. Herbal Sunscreen/UV Protection Cream Formulation:**

- **Ingredients:** These formulations incorporate botanical extracts known for sun-protective properties, such as beetroot, flax seed, green tea, papaya, aloe vera, sandalwood, tomato, chamomile, licorice root, grape seed, and shea butter. Carrier oils (e.g., avocado, almond, carrot seed, raspberry) and emulsifying agents (e.g., stearic acid, cetyl alcohol, stearyl alcohol, glycerine, triethanolamine, potassium hydroxide) are also used.
- **Procedure (Hydroalcoholic Extracts):** A sample (e.g., 10 g of beetroot, flax seed, and green tea extracts) is mixed with 60 mL distilled water and 40 mL methanol, extracted overnight, filtered, and centrifuged to yield a clear solution.

- **Procedure (Cream):** The preparation involves two phases. An aqueous phase is prepared by dissolving glycerine, potassium hydroxide, and triethanolamine in water, heating to 70°C, and then adding various plant extracts. An oil phase is prepared by melting oils, fatty alcohols, and stearic acid.

**Result:** Herbal Cosmetics (Lip Balm, Lipstick, Facial Cream, Herbal Hair and Nail Care Products) was formulated.

**References**


1. Spectrometric Identification of Organic compounds- Robert M Silverstein, 6 th edition, John Wiley & Sons,2004.
2. Principles of Instrumental Analysis- Doglas A Skoog, F. James Holler, Timothy A. Nieman, 5th edition, Eastern press, Bangalore, 1998.
3. Instrumental methods of analysis– Willards, 7th edition, CBS publishers.
4. Practical Pharmaceutical Chemistry– Beckett and Stenlake, Vol II, 4th edition, CBS Publishers, New Delhi, 1997.
5. Organic Spectroscopy- William Kemp, 3rd edition, ELBS, 1991.
6. Quantitative Analysis of Drugs in Pharmaceutical formulation- P D Sethi, rd Edition, CBS Publishers, New Delhi, 1997.
7. Pharmaceutical Analysis- Modern methods– Part B- J W Munson, Volume 11, Marcel Dekker Series
8. Pharmaceutical Technology. (2025). The role of thin-layer chromatography (TLC) and high-performance liquid chromatography (HPLC) in herbal drug analysis.
9. *Handbook of Thin-Layer Chromatography* (3rd ed.). CRC Press.
10. Research Journal of Pharmacy and Technology (RJPT). (n.d.). HPTLC method development of herbal drugs and its applications.
11. Pharmacognosy Research. Advancements in quantitative and qualitative methods for quality control of herbal drugs: A comprehensive review.
12. International Journal of Pharmacy Sciences (IJPS). (n.d.). Herbal drug formulation: Quality aspects and standards. Retrieved from
13. IOSR Journal of Pharmacy and Biological Sciences (IOSRPHR). (n.d.). Pharmacognostical evaluation of Cedrela Toona Roxb. leaves and fruits.
14. Kowalska, T. (2022). Thin-layer chromatography (TLC) in the screening of botanicals and herbal medicines. *Molecules*, 27(20), 6500. Sherma, J., & Fried, B. (2003).

www.ingramcontent.com/pod-product-compliance
Lightning Source LLC
LaVergne TN
LVHW060043210926
848481LV00013B/3947